AF556158

Infectious Diseases of Domestic Animals

Prof. S.M. Mohiuddin (Retd.)
B.V. Sc., M.V. Sc. Ph.D. (Path.)
Department of Pathology,
College of Veterinary Science,
Andhra Pradesh Agricultural University,
Rajendranagar, Hyderabad - 500 030, India

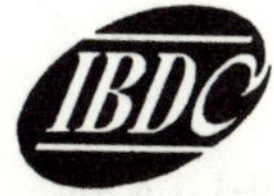

International Book Distributing Co.
(Publishing Division)

Published by

INTERNATIONAL BOOK DISTRIBUTING CO.

(Publishing Division)
Khushnuma Complex Basement
7, Meerabai Marg (Behind Jawahar Bhawan)
Lucknow 226 001 U.P. (INDIA)
Tel. : 91-522-2209542, 2209543, 2209544, 2209545
Fax : 0522-4045308
E-Mail : ibdco@airtelbroadband.in

First Edition 2007

Price: Rs.

ISBN 81-8189-122-8

Composed & Designed at :
Panacea Computers
3rd Floor, Agarwal Sabha Bhawan
Subhash Mohal,
Sadar Lucknow-226 002
Tel : 0522-2483312, 93359 27082
E-mail : prasgupt@rediffmail.com, prasgupt@hotmail.com

Printed at:
Salasar Imaging Systems
C-7/5, Lawrence Road Industrial Area
Delhi - 110 035
Tel. : 011-27185653, 9810064311

PREFACE

The Object in preparing the Book **"Infectious Diseases of domestic animals"** is to provide a comprehensive and complete important information to the under-graduate and post-graduate veterinary students. The emphasis is made to focus on the information about the actiological agents and their transmission. Pathogenises, symptoms, lesions, diagnosis and differential diagnosis have been discussed.

We hope that the information provided in this book will be useful to the students and can be easily understood and remembered in diagnosing infectious diseases.

Dr. S.M. MOHIUDDIN.

Contents

1

DISEASES CAUSED BY BACTERIA

ANTHRAX (Charban, Splenic fever)

It is an acute septicaemic disease caused by Bacillus anthrasis, gram positive capsulated, spore forming rod-shaped aerobic organism.

Transmission:

1. Infection of spores with contaminated food and water.
2. By biting files, carnivores birds, movement of infected hides, bone meal, hair and wool.
3. Inhalation of spores in man wool - saters, disease.

Incubation period : 1 to 14 days.

Pathogenesis:

1. The ingested bacilli reaches the tonsils, where they multiply and reach subsequently to lymphatic glands.
2. The bacilli are destroyed in the stomach by gastric juice.
3. The organisms contain capsule (glutamyl polypeptide), which prevents phagocytic activity on neutrophils and the clotting of blood (fibrinotytic). Thus facilitate the spread of the infection.
4. The organism becomes septicaemic a few hours before death in cattle and sheep and are only localised in horse, dog and pig.
5. The bacilli that proliferate may plug the capillaries resulting haemorrhages and the toxins produced by them also causes haemorrhages.

6. Death occurs in 12-30 hours after the onset of symptoms.
7. Spores do not form in the living animal but form when the dead body is opened. Hence the carcass should not be opened.

Symptoms:

1. They are variable and may be absent with death in peracute cases.
2. High temperature (106^{0}F).
3. Anorexia, depression, droopy ears, grinding of teeth and death in convulsions.
4. Dark coloured blood oozes from the natural orfices just before death.
5. In horses cosic is frequent.

Lesions:

1. Carcass readily undergoes purification with much gas formation.
2. The blood is dark coloured and fail to coagulate.
3. Haemorrhages on the muscular subcutaneous and serus tissues.
4. In horses, dog and pigs extensive gelatinous oedema over abdomen, thorax, limbs and external genetalia.
5. Spleenomegale in cattle, which is absent in sheep, horse, dog and swine.

Diagnosis:

1. The disease must differentiated from lightening stroke, lead poisoning and snake bite.
2. Blood smears from the ear were stained with Giemsa's reveal red capsule. And M'Fadyean Methalene blue

disintegrating capsule appear purplish blue.

3. Fluorescent antibody technique may be made use of on blood and tissues.

4. Biological test: Mice or G.Pig inoculated subcutaneously die within 36-48 hours, with gelatinous exudate at the site of inoculation. Organism may be demonstrated in blood.

5. Differenciation between:

Anthrax Bacilli and	**P.M. invaders**
a) Organism are in short chains	a) Long chains
b) Spores are absent	b) Present
c) The ends are truncated	c) Ends are round
d) Bacteria stain light	d) Stain deeply

Material for laboratory tests:

1. Smears form the ear vein or oedma fluid.
2. Muzzle for Ascolis test.

CLOSTRIDIAL INFECTION:

1. Organism of the genus clostridium are sporulating, anaerobic, gram positive.
2. They are primary cause of disease in farm animals.
3. All produce exotoxins upon which their pathogenesis depends.
4. Pathogenic clostridia are commonly present in soils rich in human and animal intestinal contents.

BLACK QUARTER

(Black leg quarter ill, symptomatic Anthrax, carbon symptomatic, Raischbrand).

It is caused by cl. chauvoei produce which an acute, highly fatal disease of cattle and occasionally of sheep, goats and swine. The organism seen as in navicular form (boat shaped) they show intensely staining at one pole while the rest of the organism is faintly stained.

Transmission:

1. Ingestion of contaminated food and water.
2. Wound infection (catastration, shearing, docking, parturition).
3. Young animals between the age of 6 months suffer more.

Incubation period : 1 to 5 days.

Pathogenesis:

1. The ingested spores are carried away by the Macrophagen across the mucosa of intestine to muscle.
2. When the muscle is devitalised by trauma or fatigue, the organims produce toxins.
3. These toxins prevent the phagocytic activity of neutrophils causing damage to endothelium leading to oedema and necrosis of muscle.
4. The organism ferment sugars in muscle and evince rancid butter smell.

Symptoms:

1. Temperature may go up to 107°F with depression and loss of appetite.
2. At the point of entry of organisms the skin appear purplish, and oedema of subcutaneous tissue.
3. There is no cripitation, but pits on presence.
4. If the lesions are on leg it laments more.
5. If the lesions are in genital tract there is stiffness and staggering gait.

Lesions:

1. When the lesion is cut open serosanguinous, foul smelling fluid may exude.
2. Affected muscle is dark red, dry and spongy.
3. Such lesions are noticed in heart, kidneys, spleen and lungs.
4. Fibrinous, Haemorrhagic pericarditis, pluracy and endocarditis.

HOSTOPATHOLOGY:

Muscle showed waxy degeneration and coagulative necrosis, cross straition are retained with haemorrhages and oedema between the fillers.

Diagnosis:

1. Demonstration of organism form the lesions.
2. Characteristic lesions.
3. G. Pig inoculation-infected material inoculated into the thigh muscle. The animal dies after 48 hours with characteristic lesions.

MALIGNANT OEDMA

(Grass gangreen)

Primarily caused by cl. Septicum but frequently associated with cl.ch.auvei, cl. novyi, cl.perfringens, and cl. sporogens.

Transmission:

1. Malignant oedema is seen as a sequal to wound infection (shearing, docking, parturition, vaccination).
2. It is frequent in horses, sheep and cattle, but rare in dogs and cats.

Pathogenesis:

Organisms produce powerful toxin, which inhibit the activity of neutraphils, injures capillary endothelium, thus causing oedema and necrosis of muscle fibers. Organisms ferment glycogen producing gas.

Symptoms:

1. Short febrile course with a hot, painful swelling at the site of infection.
2. Death within 24-48 hours.
3. Creptating and crackling sound. Frothy blood tinged exudate may be discharged from the wound.

Lesions:

1. The skin on the affected area is gangrenous, cold and bluish.
2. Cl. chauvei produce typical muscle lesion as seen in B.Q.
3. Cl.pefringens produce haemorrhagic oedma with gangrene.
4. Cl. Novei produce excessive clear gelatinous oedema without haemorrhages or gas.

Diagnosis:

1. Based on symptoms and lesions.
2. Demonstration of the organism.

BRAXY

BRODSOT

It is an acute toxemic and fatal disease of weaning lambs and yearlings. It is caused by cl.septicum. This disease is always associated with infectious necrotic hepatitis and enterotoxemia.

Transmission:

1. Eating frosty grass during winter pre-disposes the animals to infection.
2. Usually animals in good health are affected.

Symptoms:

1. Not usually noticed and often the lambs were found dead in the morning.
2. Depression, abdominal pain and diarrhoea.
3. Affected animals stand aloof from others and grinding of teeth is common.
4. Abdomen is bloated.
5. Death occurs within few hours.

Lesions:

1. The wall of the abomassum is edimus and haemorrhagic.
2. Similar lesion may be seen in small intestine.
3. The peritonial and pericardial cavities contain fluid.
4. Kidneys and liver showed toxic changes.

Diagnosis:

1. Based on history and lesions.
2. The organism can be demonstrated in tissues.

BLACK DISEASE :

(Infectious Necrotic Hepatitis)

It is an acute fatal infection of sheep and rarely cattle. It is caused by cl.novyi (cl.oedematieus) type B.

Transmission:

1. The organisms are widely distributed in soil as type ABC passes through intestinal wall and lodge in the liver and remain as patient infection.
2. An anaerobic environment is produced by the migration of liver fluke (Fasiola hepatica, Dicrocoelium dendriticum).
3. The parasitic infection activates the bacteria, which releases

endotoxins further contributing to hepatic necrosis and fatal toxemia.

Symptoms:

A. Animals are dull, lag behind the flock and die without struggling.

Lesions:

1. Dark appearance of the flesh on side of the felt due to extensive subcutaneous haemorrhages hence the name Black disease.
2. Hydropricardium with clear fluid is characteristic.
3. Thoracic and abdominal cavities contain excess of fluid.
4. Liver is dark due to engorgement with necrotic foci mostly on diapharmatic lobe.

Histopathology:

1. Liver showed scars due to the migration of immature flukes.
2. The pyloric region of the stomach shows congested mucosa and clear gelatinous oedema in submucosa.

Diagnosis:

1. Lesions and histopathological changes.
2. Demonstration of organism in the liver impression smears.

BOVINE BACILLARY HAEMOGDOBINURIA

It is caused by cl.haemolyticum cattle mostly affected.

Transmission:

1. The organism present in low lying swampy areas.
2. Spores also found in bones of carcasses upto 2 years.

Lesions:

1. Liver contains large areas of infacts as a constant feature.

2. Serous cavities contain blood stained fluid.
3. Haemorrhages on the peritonium and pericardium are constant.

Diagnosis:

1. Based on pathological findings and isolation of organism.

ENTEROTOXEMIA

(Pulpy kidney disease, overeating disease).

It is an acute toxemia of sheep of all ages, but mostly of lambs. It is caused by cl. perfringens type-D.

Transmission:

1. The organism are the normal inhabitant of intestinal tract.
2. When animals were fed with starchy diet and associated with impaction.
3. In fattening sheep maintained in high nutrition diet.

Symptoms:

1. Morbidity is low and mortality is high (100%).
2. The toxin produced consist of epsilon which causes diarrohea convulsions and optsthotonus.
3. Sheep that survive, keep themselves aloof, depressed with drooping head, staggers with champing of jaws and salivation.
4. The animal walks in circles.
5. Head pressing against hard objects.

Lesions:

1. Petechial haemorrhages beneath the epicardium, endocardial surface, the serosa of intestine, abdominal muscles, diaphragm, and thymus.

2. Hydropericardium with straw coloured fluid.
3. Pronounced glycosuria.
4. Softening of kidney-pulpy kidney.
5. In brain lysis and liquification of white matter while the grey matter is oedematus.

In addition to the classical type-D enterotoxemia, cl.perfringens type A, B and C cause enterotoxemia in animals.

Cl.perfringens type A:

1. Lambs and calves affected with a short course and high mortality.
2. Intense icterus and haemolytic anaemia with haemoglobin urea.
3. Icterus, anaemia, excess pericardial fluid, dark kidneys and enlarged friable liver.

Cl. perfringence Type B. (Lam dysentry):

1. Lambs less than two weeks age are affected.
2. Reluctant to suckle, lying down and exhibit signs of pain.
3. Faeces semifluid, brownish and contain blood.
4. Haemorrhagic enteritis-with ulcers is a characteristic lesion.

Cl. perfringence type C:

Two distinct forms of enterotoxemia are produced:-

A. Struck:

1. Affects adult sheep.
2. Haemorrhagic enteritis with ulceration of mucosa from deuodenum and jejunum.

B. Enterotoxic haemorrhagic enteritis:

1. Affects calves and lambs in first few days of life.

2. Haemorrhagic enteritis with ulcers.

Diagnosis:

1. Lesions are diagnostic.
2. Demonstration of cl.perfringence toxins in the intestinal contents by neutralization test in mice.
3. Rabbit inoculation with intestinal toxins dies in few minutes to hours.

TETANUS

(Lock jaw)

It is a highly fatal infectious disease caused by the cl. teatni. It is world wide.

Transmission:

1. The organism are widely distributed in cultivated soil.
2. Infection is always wound contamination following docking, shearing, castration and vaccination.
3. Incubation period is 1-2 weeks.

Pathogenesis:

1. Spores entering wound vegitate and liberate two types of toxins viz. a) haemohysin b) tetanospasmin.
2. Haemolysis is responsible for haemolysis.
3. Tetanospasmin—absorbed by the axons of the peripheral nerves to spinal cord and brain—causes hyperirritability and tetanic spasums.

Symptoms:

1. Locked jaw—the muscles of the jaw are firmly contracted.
2. Stiffness of limbs with straddling gait (swash back attitude).
3. Arched back, errect tail, and neck opisthotonus.

4. The animal has anxious looks and paralysis of membrane nictitans.
5. Respiration laboured.
6. Temperature remains normal but increases just before death.
7. When face is raised the eyes are completely closed.

Lesions:

1. Blood is black and tarry colour.
2. Rigor mortis sets in immediately.
3. Haemorrhages seen on muscles.
4. Wounds have a bad odour due to putrifaction.

Diagnosis:

1. Symptoms are diagnostic.
2. Organism can be demonstrated in the smears prepared from deep seats of wound.

BOTULISM
(LAMB SICKNESS)

It is a fatal intoxication by the toxins of cl.botulinum.

Transmission:

1. The organisms are normal inhabitant of digestive tract.
2. The organisms propagate on carcases, bones, rotting vegetables in warm and moist atmosphere.
3. Incubation period is 12 hours to 3 days.

Symptoms:

1. Paralysis of skeletal muscles—Neurotoxin is produced by the organism and prevents the formation of acetylcholene at parasympathetic and skeletal motor nerve endings.

2. Paralysis of pharynx, tongue and limb.
3. The head droops and incoordinating movement.
4. Respiration is shallow and abdominal.

Lesions:

1. Not characteristic, however haemorrhages in epicardium, endocardium and neurons degeneration.

Diagnosis:

1. Symptoms are diagnostic.
2. Filtrates of suspected feed injected to G.Pig and mice die of paralysis.

PASTEURLOSIS

(Haemorrhagic Septicemia, shipping fever)

It is an acute septicemic disease of animals, caused by short gram negative non-motile organisms. High fever, depression, multiple haemorrhages, pneumonia, pericarditis and arthritis are characteristic features.

Transmission :

1. Ingestion of contaminated food and water.
2. Organisms are natural inhabitant of tonsils and nasopharynx. Invade the tissues when the resistance of the animal is reduced (fatigue, starvation, confined to humid and dampness).

Symptoms:

1. High fever 104-107°F.
2. Prostration, diarrhoea, weakness of head, mucosal discharges from eye and nose.
3. Death occurring in 24 hours.
4. Frequent coughing and grunting.

5. In latter stages lameness develops in one or more limbs.

Lesions:

1. Swelling of head, neck and throat.
2. Petechae on all serous and mucous membranes, especially on the endocardium, peritoneum, pleura and gastro-intestinal tract.
3. Fibrinous broncho-pneumonia. The interlobular septa is thickned and infiltrated with serus fluid producing marbling.
4. Fibrinous pluracy.
5. Lymphatic glands swollen and haemorrhagic.

Diagnosis:

1. Symptoms and lesions are diagnostic.
2. Demonstration of bipolar organims in blood.
3. Rabbit inoculation with infective material dies within 48 hours with haemorrhagic tracheitis.

Paratyphoid in Animals

(Salmonellosis)

Many species of antigenetically related organisms are found in the genus salmonella. They are gram negative and rod shaped. The organisms are classified based upon identification of the antigen in the cell was (O" antigen) and flagella (H" antigen). The commonest species that are associated with disease in man and animals are.

	Organims	**Hosts**	**Disease**
1	S.Cholerae-suis	Swine	Enteritis, septicemia
2	S.Typhi (Bacterium Typhi, Eberthella type)	Man	Typhoid fever
3	S. Paralyphi-A	Man	Paratyphoid-A

	Organims	Hosts	Disease
4	S. Schottmue thesi (Bacterium paratyphoid-B, B.Schottmuellari)	Man, rarely animals	Enteric fever paratyphoid-B
5	S.Typhimurium	Rodents, many other animals & man	Gastroeneritis
6	S.enteritidis	Man and other species	Enteritis
7	S.gallinarum	Poultry	Enteritis septicemia fowl poisioning
8	S.give	Cattle	Enteritis
9	S.pullorum	Chicks	Enteritis, septicemia pullorim disease
10	S.abortus equi	Horse	Abortion
11	S.dublin	Cattle, swine sheep	Abortion, enteritis septicemia, osteomyelitis, meningitis.
12	S.anatum	Ducks, monkeys	Enteritis, septicemia

Transmission:

1. Contaminated food and water.
2. Young ones are more susceptible.
3. Recovered animals remain as carriers (infection localises in liver, spleen, mesenertic lymph nodes and gall bladder) excrete through faeces.
4. Salmonellae from birds and animals are responsible for "food poisoning" in man.

Symptoms:

Are classified according to severity in four groups.

A. ***Septicemia:***

1. New born calves, fowls and young pigs upto 4 months are commonly affected.
2. Depression, dullness, high fever (105-107°F) and death within 24-48 hours.
3. Calves show incoordination and nystagmus.
4. Pigs—dark red to purple colour of the skin, abdomen, ears and subcutanous petechial haemorrhages.
5. Mortality rate is 100%.

B. Acute enteritis:

1. Common in all adult animals.
2. High temperature (104-106°F) with severe watery diarrhoea.
3. The faeces is feetid smell and contain mucous.
4. Mortality rate is 75%.

C. Sub-acute enteritis:

1. Mostly common in horses.
2. Faeces consistency is of cow manure.

D. Chronic enteritis:

1. Persistant diarrhoea.
2. Intermittant fever with emaciation.
3. The faeces contain spots of blood, mucous and firm at intervals.

Lesions:

They are enterocolitis and septecemic.

1. The lesion are seen commencing in the ileum and extending to colon, mucosa is hypermic, thickened, often covered with a red, yellow, or grey exudate and ulcers. There are no lesions in stomach and proximal intestine.
2. Small foci of necrosis (typhoid nodules) in the liver.
3. Hyperplasia of lymph nodes and spleen.
4. In septicemic form, fibrinodi necrosis of vessel wall and hyaline material deposits in glomerular capillaries are noticed.
5. Rectal structures in swine following prolonged ulcerative proctitis.
6. Abortion occurs between 6-9 month of gestation.
7. Ediema, focal haemorrhages and necrosis found on placenta and foetus.

Diagnosis:

1. Based on symptoms and lesions.
2. Isolation of organisms is necessary for confirmation.
3. Immunofluorescence method.

LISTERIOSIS (CIRCLING DISEASE)

Listeriosis is responsible for abortion in man, cattle, sheep and goats. Meningeal or encephalitic infection in man, cattle, sheep goat and swine and systemic (septicemic) infection in man, cattle sheep, swine, dogs, cats. Rodents are reserviors. The organisms are small, rod shaped, gram positive, non-sporulating and motile, mortaliy is 100% and morbidity 10%.

Transmission:

1. Infection through contaminated food and water.
2. Infected animals discharge infection through faeces, urine, aborted foetuses, uterine discharges, and in milk.

3. Nervous form of infection occurs, through nasal mucosa or conjunctiva.
4. Infection through coitus.

Pathogenesis:

The organisms penetrate the epithelial cells conjunctive, urinary bladder, and intestine and multiply, destroy the cells and are released to be phagocytised by macrophages resulting in septicemia. Then they localise in different organs.

Symptoms:

This can be studied under

A. Listerial Menningeo Encephalitis:-

1. The disease is more acute in sheep than cattle. Death occurs in 3-4 days in sheep than cattle.
2. High temperature with associated symptoms.
3. The neck is pulled to one side and moves in circle—hence the name circling diseases.
4. Head is pressed against fixed objects.
5. Prehension and mastication are slow with drooling of saliva for long periods.
6. Unilateral paralysis—ear, eye lids and lips.
7. Infection in early pregnancy, results in abortion and in late still births.

B. Septicemic Listeriosis (visceral form):-

1. Common in monogastric young animals, fowl, young pigs, newborn lambs and calves.
2. Lack of nervous symptoms.
3. Symptoms associated with gastro-enteritis and hepatic necrosis.
4. Corneal opacity with dyspnoea, nystagmus and mild opisthotonus.

5. Death in 12 hours.

C. Abortion:

1. Infection in early pregnancy, results in abortion and in late still births.
2. Delivery of young rapidly develops a fatal septicaemia.

Lesions:

A. Encephalitis:

1. Microbacess associated with mononuclear cells infiltration. Lesions in brain stem, medulla elangata and spinal cord.
2. Visceral lesions similar to those seen septicemic form may also be noticed.

B. Şepticemia (visceral form):

1. Focal necrosis of liver and less frequently of spleen, lymphnodules, lungs, adrenal glands, myocardium, gastro-intestinal tract.
2. In birds—death is sudden, massive, cardiac necrosis, pericarditis with increased pericardial fluid.
3. Liver enlarged, friable with necrotic foci.
4. Fibrinous peritonitis and enteritis.
5. Spleen enlarged.

C. Abortion:

1. Focal liver cell necrosis of aborted foetus containing stainable organisms.

Diagnosis:

1. Symptoms and lesions.
2. Demonstration of organims in tissues and isolation of organisms.

3. Biological test: Rabbit when inoculated with infected material into the eye, conjunctivitis results. Intraceranial inoculation results in death in 2-3 days.
4. Fluorescent antibody test.

BRUCELLOSIS (BANGAS DISEASE)

(Contagious abortion)

It is caused by different strains of Brucellia a gram negative small bacilli in livestock and man.

Diseases caused by different species:

a) Br. Aborttus - Abortion in cattle and infertility in bulls.

b) Br. Ovis - Abortion in sheep and infertility in rams.

c) Br. Melitensis in rams - Abortion and sterility in goats. Gastric fever, Malta fever or Mediterranean fever in man.

d) Br. Swiss - Sterility and abortion in sows architis in boar.

e) Br. Bronchiseptica - Associated with chronic pneumonia in piglets and calves.

Transmission:

1. Through contaminated food and water, aborted foetus, foetal membrane discharges from uterus, and milk from affected animals.
2. Through coitus from an infected bull.
3. Contamination of udder during milking.

Incubation period: Variable between 1 month to 8 months.

Pathogenesis:

The organism has a prediliction for pregnant uterus, udder, testis, male sexglands, lymphnodes, joint capsule and bursa. After the initial invasion of the body localisation occurs in tissues and attracts phagocytic cells and multiply in these cells with predominant accumulation of epitheliod cells resulting in a nodule.

Symptoms:

1. Abortion after 5th month of pregnancy is the cardinal sign.
2. Second or even third abortion occur followed by full term pregnancy.
3. Retention of placenta and mastitis is common.
4. Architis and epidirimitis.
5. Enlarged seminal vesicles.
6. Affected males are sterile.
7. In swine lameness, inco-ordination and posterior paralysis are most common.

Lesions:

1. Placental lesion (a) early stage - cotyledons are dull, granular in appearance and intercotiledonary chorion is oedimatus (b) advance stages, yellowish granular necrotic areas on the surface of the foetal cotyledon and the rest of the chorion is opaque, thick and leathery in consistency.
2. In swine the infected uterine mucosa bears tiny white to yellowish nodules.
3. In males orchitis with enlarged and indurated sex organs.
4. Liver spleen and lymphatic glands are swollen, hyperimic with necrotic foci.

Diagnosis:

1. Symptoms and lesions.
2. Demonstration of organisms from the lesions.
3. G.Pig inoculation for isolation of organisms.
4. Agglutination test with serum milk, vaginal mucosa and seminal plasma.

5. A.B.R. (Abortus bang ring) test: One drop of coloured antigen mixed with one ml of fresh milk in a sterile test tube. In positive cases a ring will form.

VIBRIOSIS (VIBRIONIC ABORTION)

Campylobacteriosis.

The organisms are responsible for abortion and infertility in cattle. The organisms are gram negative, comma or "S" shaped and motile (flagilla lophotichus).

Transmission:

1. Contaminated food and water.
2. Coital infection as organisms do not multiply in intestinal tract.

Pathogenesis:

1. The placenta of pregnant animals is invaded by organisms, becomes necrotic and separated.
2. There will be endometritis, cervicitis and vaginitis.

Symptoms:

1. Temporary infertility and prolonged oestrus.
2. Abortion in late pregnancy (4 months).
3. Males are not affected.
4. In sheep late abortion, still births or birth of week lambs which usually die soon after birth.

Lesions:

1. Mucopurulent endometritis.
2. In sheep the cotyledons are swollen, soft, congested with grey areas of necrosis.
3. Oedema of the serus cavities and peritonial tissues in the foetus.

4. Foetal liver showed necrotic foci.

Diagnosis:

1. Demonstration of the organism in the discharges and in the lesions.
2. Agglutination test with cervical mucosa.
3. Fluorescence antibody test on cervical mucosa.

SWINE ERYSIPELES

It is an infectious disease of pigs characterised by diamond- shaped skin lesions in acute form and non-supportive arthritis, vegetative endocarditis in chronic form. The organisms are Erysipelothrix rhusiopathiae (E.insidiosa) is small pleomorphic rod- shaped either straight or curved gram positive and intraleucocytic. Cattle and sheep are rarely affected. Man is susceptible. Young pigs 3-6 months old are mostly susceptible. Recovered animals are carriers.

Transmission:

1. Contaminated food and water through infected faeces.
2. Fleas are known to transmit.
3. Through skin abrations.

Pathogenesis:

1. The organisms gain entry into the circulation through tonsils and intestine and multiply resulting septicemia.
2. Bacilli that enter through skin wounds reach blood through lymph.
3. The organisms liberates toxins which injures the blood vessel wall resulting in erythematus lesions.
4. In few cases the organisms localises in the skin causing thrombosis of the small vessels, leading to diamond lesions.

Symptoms:

A. Acute form :

1. Incubation period is 1-7 days with 75% mortality.
2. High temperature upto 108°F.
3. Skin lesions—Characteristic diamond-shaped, red utricarial plaques, diffuse Oedematus Peruptons (diamond skin disease), common on belly, inside the thigh, on throat, neck and ears.

B. Chronic form:

1. Arthritis—characteristic due to localisation of organisms in elbow, hip hock, stiffle and knee joints leading to lameness.
2. Hyperkeratosis of back, shoulder and leg regions.
3. Alopecia and sloughing of the tail, tip of the ears.
4. Endocarditis with concomitant symptoms is constant.

Lesions:

A. Acute form:

1. Diamond skin lesions.
2. Ecchymotic haemorrhages throughout the body, plura, peritonium, under the kidney capsule.
3. Infarcts in the spleen and kidneys.
4. Liver enlarged and congested.
5. Lungs oedematus.

B. Chronic form: Non-suppurative arthitis.

1. Joint enlarged, thickened and distended with excessive fluid.
2. Heart endocarditis—large irregularly course masses.
3. Articular cartilage may ulcerate.
4. Ankylosis may supervene leading to lameness.

Diagnosis:

1. Symptoms and lesions.
2. Demonstration of organisms in blood during septecemic stage.
3. White mice die in 12 hours of inoculation of infection and the organisms can be demonstrated in spleen.

CASEOUS LYMPHADENITIS

(Pseudotuberculosis of sheep)

Is a chronic disease of sheep and goats, caused by corynebacterium pseudotuberculosis (cerynebacterim ovis) a gram positive diptheroid bacilli.

Transmission:

1. Always wound infection-docking, shearing and castration wounds.
2. Unhealed umbalicus.
3. In few cases through contaminated feed and water.

Pathogensis:

1. The organisms from the local areas are transported by macropahges to the regional lymphnodes.
2. Necrosis of the paranchma due to exotoxins produced by the organisms.
3. The necrotic foci coagulaised becomes liquified and encapsulated and forms abscess.
4. The organisms gain entrance into lung, liver, kidney and produce microabscess.

Symptoms:

1. Enlargement of superificial lymphnodes (submaxillas, precapsular, prefemoral, supramammary and popliteal).

2. Respiratory symptoms when lungs are involved.
3. Urinary symptoms pyelonephritis.

Lesions:

1. Lymphatic glands show concentricaly lamillated layers of fibrous capsule alternating with caseous firm material that may be green and occasionally gritty, and giving onion skin appearance.
2. Lungs abscess.
3. Kidneys showed pyelonephritis.

Diagnosis:

1. Lesions
2. Demonstration of organism in pus.
3. Biological test—G. Pig inoculated with infected material die in 4-10 days with caseous nodules in liver, associated lymph nodes and lungs.

BOTRIOMYCOSIS

A granulomatus lesion caused by staphylococcus aureus. It is frequent in horses as wound contamination. The lesion is of dense granulation tissue with abscess in the centre. It is connected to the skin with sinus. Organisms present in the pus.

In calves and pigs the mammary gland is usually affected with chronic mastitis.

Lesions:

A granuloma with a dense granulation tissue in the centre which latter form abscess. Metastasis for the primary lesion may occur in the regional lymphodes and also in internal organs.

COLIBACILLOSIS

Is a disease of newborn animals of all species, caused by the E.coli a gram negative rod-shaped organisms.

The different strains of Escherichia coli have ability under certain conditions of host, produces pathological changes involving at least four pathogenic mechanisms.

A) " ENTEROTOXIC COLIBACILLOSIS":

Common in young piglets, calves and lambs. The organisms adhere to the mucosa and proliferate in the lumen of small intestine, producing a potent endotoxin which causes excessive secretion of fluid from the intestinal mucosa. This loss of fluid causes diarrhoea, dehydration and death.

B) ENTEROTOXEMIC COLIBACILLOSIS:

(Enterotoximic colibaccillosis of calves and edema disease of swine)

The organisms grow in the small intestine producing toxins that is absorbed and acts elsewhere. This toxin is different from enterotoxin and is a neurotoxin (oedema disease principle). In swine this form is manifested by oedema of gastric, colonic, palfbebral, subcutaneous and central nervous tissues.

C) SEPTICEMIC COLIBACILLOSIS:

Seen mostly in young calves. The organisms invade the host through oral cavity, respiratory system, pharynx or umbalicus and produce endotoxin which causes the lesions. Diarrhoea and intestinal lesions are absent.

D) LOCAL INVASIVE COLIBACILLOSIS:

Mostly seen in man. The organisms invade the epithelium of colon and produce lesions-dysentery, fever and multiple foci of ulcerative enteritis.

TUBERCULOSIS:

The disease is caused by Mycobacterium tuberculosis, organisms small acid fast bacilli. These organisms occur as pairs lying at an angle pole to pole or arranged in bundle of faggets. The disease is characterised by progressive development of tubercles in various organs in different species.

Species susceptability:

The organisms are classified in species as M.Bovis. M. Avim and M.Tubercolosis.

Species - Type :

1. Man - Human and bovine
2. Horse - Bovine and rarely with avian.
3. Cattle - Bovine and rarely with avian and human
4. Sheep and goats - Bovine human and avian.
5. Pigs - Bovine, avian and human.
6. Dogs - human and bovine.
7. Poultry - Avain.

Susceptibility of laboratory animals

Type	G.Pig	Rabbit	Fowl
Human	+ +	+	-
Bovine	+ + +	+ +	-
Avian	-	+ +	+

Transmission:

1. Organisms are excreted in the exhaled air, sputum, faeces, milk, urine, vaginal and uterine discharges with contaminated food and water.
2. Inhalation.
3. Less common routes intrauterine infection through infected bull and intramammary through contaminated milk machines.
4. Congenital infection is associated with tuberculosis metritis.

Incubation period: 6-12 months.

Pathogenesis:

Tuberculosis spreads in the body by way of :

a) Primary complex.

b) Post-primary dissemination .

Primary complex:

1. Lesions are present at the point of entry of infection and in local lymphnodes.
2. This is common when infection is by inhalation.
3. Primary lesion is mostly in diaphragmatic lobe of lungs and spreads through lymphites leading to pneumonia.
4. Sometimes these organisms are coughed up and then swallowed, then resulting secondary infection in digestive system.

Post-primary dissemination

1. It varies considerably in rate and route.
2. It may result as miliary tuberculosis-discrete nodular lesions in various organs.
3. Chronic organ tuberculosis.
4. Chronic organ tuberculosis caused by endogenous or exogenous reinfection of tissues rendered allergic to tuberculoprotein.
5. In the latter case there may not be involvement of local lymph nodules.
6. Depending upon the site of localisation of infection, clinical signs vary, but there is constant toxaemia.

The ingested bacilli are engulfed by macrophages (epitheliod cells). If the cells are not destroyed, these bacilli multiply and released thus engulfed by other macrophages. The centre of the lesion becomes caseous due to accumulation of necrotic macrophages. As the tuberculosis bacilli multiply and produce toxic substances, the adjacent cells undergo caseous necrosis and more epitheloid granulation tissue is laid down around the caseous centre. The cells making up the granulation tissue have abundant foamy, pale acidophilic cytoplasm and round often that excentrically placed nuclei. These cells may coalesce to form langhans giant cells. The granulation tissue is usually surrounded by a zone of lymphocytes. As the lesion ages, it is encapsulated with a connective tissue. Classification of caseous centre occurs, in all species except birds.

Symptoms:

Symptoms are associated with involvement of system.

Cattle:

1. Chronic cough due to broncho-pneumonia which can never be loud.
2. Dyspnoea with increased rate and depth of respiration.
3. Tuberculous lesions of small intestine causes diarrhoea.
4. Painless swelling of submaxilly prescapular, prescapular, suprammary lymphnodes.
5. Tuberculous architis is characterised by large endurated painless testis.
6. Tuberculous mastitis—marked induration, hypertrophy of udder.

Pigs:

1. Symptoms as in cattle.
2. Involvment of meninges and joints are more common.

Horses:

1. Stiffness of the neck due to Osteomyelitis of cervical vertebrae.

2. Other symptom as in cattle.

Sheep and goat—Same as cattle.

Lesions:

1. Tuberculous granulomas may be found in all the affected organs and lymphatic glands.
2. In lungs miliary abscess containing creamy to orange coloured pus.
3. Ulcers in intestine and payers patches.
4. Ostemyclitis in bones.

Diagnosis:

1. Symptoms and lesions.
2. Tuberculin test.
3. Demonstration of organism in milk.
4. G. Pig inoculated with suspected material subscutaneously in the thigh tuberculus lesion will be seen after 6-7 weeks on necropsy.

JHONE'S DISEASE

(Paratuberculosis)

It is a chronic wasting disease of ruminants, rarely horse and pigs are affected. It is characterised by chronic enteritis. The disease is caused by mycobacteria paratuberculosis an acid-fast organism similar to that of tuberculous baccili.

Incubation period: 2 years.

Transmission:

1. Contaminated feed and water with faeces of infected animals.

Symptoms:

1. Diarrhoea which is neither offensive nor blood stained.

2. Faeces is soft.
3. Inspite of good appetite and feeding the animal progressively, it becomes weak and emaciated with increasing thirst.
4. Sheep-Diarrhoea is not a constant symptom.

Lesions:

1. Terminal part of the ileum is the most common site, however the remainder of the small and large intestine and mesentric nodes affected.
2. Affected intestinal wall is thickned, oedematus and its mucosal surface bears many folds closely placed transverse folds giving the surface corrugated appearance.
3. These folds do not disappear when the intestinal wall is stretched.
4. Mesentric lymphodes enlarged and juicy.
5. Mesentric lymphnodes in sheep and goats are knotty.

Diagnosis:

1. Symptoms and lesions.
2. Examination of bowel washing for organisms.
3. Examination of rectal pinch for organism.
4. Johnin test.

NECROBACILLOSIS

Anaerobic, non-sporulating, gram negative filamentous organisms spherophorus, necrophorus (Fusiformis necrophorus, Fusibacterim necrophorus) are responsible for various disease conditions in following animals:

Cattle and sheep	-	Necrosis of liver
Calves	-	Calf diphtheria
Horses	-	Quittor, polevil, fistulus withers.

Fowls	-	Intestinal ulcers.
Swine	-	Necrosis of snout and tongue and other parts of body.

Transmission:

1. Organisms are ubiquitous.
2. Predisposing factors required for the disease to occur.

A) NECOVBACILLOSIS OF LIVER:

1. Liver involvement is associated with concomittant symptoms viz. fever, vomiting, anorexia and depression.
2. Liver enlarged with multiple abscess.
3. In young one omphalophlebititis is usually present.

B) CALF DIPHTHERIASIS

1. Usually calf under 6 months of age suffer.
2. Elevated tenacious necrotic plaques of larynx, pharynx and trachea.
3. Severe inspiratory dyspnoea.
4. Breath has a most foul, rancid smell.
5. Spread to lungs causing severe suppurative bronchopneumonia.

Pathogensis:

1. They cause coagulative necrosis at the point of entry, subsequently secondary bacterial infection aggrevate necrosis. Such necrotic masses are found on tongue, inside neck, gums, palate and pharynx. These lesions are covered with a dry membrane, when removed will be seen.

C) NECROTIC RHINITIS

Injury to the face, nasal cavity and oral cavity leads to this condition. Necrotic cellulitis of the soft tissues of the nose and face may spread to bones. In all the internal organs, the organism causes, necrosis thus resulting inflammation of different organs.

ACTINOBACILLOSIS

(Wooden Tongue)

It is caused by Actinobacillus ligneresi, a small non-motile, rod-shaped gram negative aerobic organism. It is characterised by granulomatus inflammation of tongue in cattle and soft tissues of head and neck in sheep.

Transmission:

1. Injury to the buccal mucosa permit the entry of the organisms.
2. Contaminated pasture feed with discharges from abscess in the mouth and regional lymphnodes.

Symptoms and lesions:

1. Excessive salivation and gentle chewing of the tongue.
2. Partially protruded immobile tongue.
3. The base of the tongue is swollen and hard but the tip is normal (wooden tongue).
4. Nodules and ulcers on the sides of the tongue and ulcers on the dorsum of the tips of tongue.
5. Lymphadinitis (submaxillary and partid) with abscess formation and discharging non-odorus pus.
6. In liver, lungs, stomach, and intestine the abscess are very small.
7. In sheep the tongue is not affected.
8. Pigs—the lesions are similar to that of cattle.
9. Microscopically, the lesions consist of discrete colonies or organisms, surrounded by radiating clubs, suspended in pus and encapsulated with connective tissue. The colonies tend to be much smaller, the radiating clubs longer and more

slender and the purulent exudate more abundant than in Actinomycosis grams—staining of the smears of section reveals gram negative organisms in the centre of the colonies, but if is difficult to detect because of the acidophilic staining of the background.

Diagnosis:

1. Characteristic lesions.
2. Demonstration of organisms in pus smear.
3. Characteristic histopathological changes.

ACTINOMYCOSIS

(Lumpy Jaw)

It is caused by gram positive rod-shaped or long filamentous organisms which are often headed and occasionally branched. The disease is most common in cattle. The organisms are associated with Br.Abortus in equine fistulous withers.

Transmission:

1. In cattle- supporting ostiomyelitis of mandible and Maxilla.
2. The swelling is hard, immovable and painful to touch.
3. The cut surface of the lesion usually is white and glistening from the dense connective tissue in which small abscesses are embedded.
4. Yellow pus form the absceses contain tiny hard masses-sulfur granules.
5. Histologically the centre of the granule contain gram positive organisms, surrounding this by a zone of radially arranged Indian clubs. Beyond this there is a zone of neutrophils surrounded by an outer area of large mononuclear (epitheliod) cells with abundant foamy cytoplasm, covered by a dense connective tissue layer.

Diagnosis:

1. Characteristic lesions.
2. Demonstration organisms in pus.
3. Characteristic histological changes.
4. Differential diagnosis between Actinobacillosis and Actinomycosis.

Actinobacillosis	Actinomycosis
1. Affects soft tissues generally	1. Affects hard tissues (bones)
2. Granules in pus is soft	2. Granules often calcified, gritty larger and darker.
3. Granules contain G - ve organisms	3. Granules contain G + organisms
4. Spreads through lymphatics	4. Spread through blood stream

GLANDERS

It is caused by pseudomonas mallei (Malleomyces mallei, Loefferella mallei, Pfeiferlla mallei, Bacillus mallei, actino bacillus mallei), a short, rod-shaped with rounded ends, gram negative organism. The disease in horses is chronic and in mules and donkeys runs on acute course.

Transmission:

1. Through inhalation.
2. Ingestion of contaminated food and water.

Symptoms:

1. The respiratory tract and lungs are mostly affected.
2. Catarrhal copious and persistant nasal discharge later becomes purulent.

3. Ulceration in nasal mucosa.
4. Chronic cough.
5. Skin lesions (Farcy)—ulcers of the skin, thickening of the superficial lymphatic gland have abscess formation.

Lesions:

1. Deep ulceration of nasal septum on healing leaves star-shaped scar.
2. Lungs show discrete granulomatus nodules with caseous necrotic centre surrounded by epitheloid cells, few giant cells and lymphocytes.
3. Such granulomas occur in liver, spleen and other viscera.
4. Skin lesion—frequent on legs, persistant ulcers connected by tortuous, indurated thick walled lymphatics—farcy.
5. Superficial lymph nodes showed suppurating and discharging thick tenacious pus.

Diagnosis:

1. Symptoms and lesions.
2. Demonstration of organisms in lesions.
3. Intraperitonial inoculation of infected material into male pig (straus test) result in acute purulent orchitis in 3-4 days. The organisms can be isolated in pure culture from the lesions.

STRANGLES

It is an infectious respiratory disease of young horses characterised by sudden onset of fever catarrh in the upper respiratory tract followed by acute swelling and abscess formation in submaxillary, parapharyngeal and other lymph nodes. It is caused by streptococcus equi organism.

Lesion:

1. Submaxillary lymph nodes enlarged, hot and firm abscess containing large quantities of yellowish pus.
2. Metastatic abscesses occur in lungs, liver, kidneys, spleen and occasionally the brain.

Diagnosis:

1. Symptoms and lesions.
2. Demonstration of organism.

EPIZOOTIC LYMPHANGITIS

It is a chronic disease affecting skin and superificial lymphatics of horses. It is caused by mycotic organisms—histoplasms-farciminosum, a gram positive cocci with double walls.

Transmission:

1. Wound infection.

Lesions:

1. Chronic indurative ulceration of skin especially of limb.
2. Thickening of superficial lymphatics, enlargement of regional lymph nodes, formation of abscess and discharging of pus.
3. Histologically the lesion reveal granulomatus changes with predominant macrophages. The central mass of fungus stained with haematoxilin, while the wall is stained with PVS stain.

Diagnosis:

1. Characteristic lesions.
2. The organism can be demonstrated in the lesions.
3. D.I.D test with cryptococcin.

LEPTOSPIROSIS

(Weils disease, stuctgart disease)

The disease occurs in dog and domestic animals caused by several species of leptospira. The spiral organisms are single, flexuous and helical with curved ends and motile by means of axial filaments (axistyle). They are best visualised under dark field microscopy and can be stained with silver impregnation method.

Disease due to Leptospira

Serotype	Species	Disease
1. L. Icterohemorrhagicae	Man, rat, dog, cattle	Weil's disease (Man) leutospirosis (Animals
2. L. Canicola	Dog, man, cattle	Leptospirosis (Animals) Haemoglobinaema (cattle) canieola fever (Man)
3. L. Pomona	Swine, cattle, sheep, man, horse	Abortion, stillbirth (swine). abortion, mastitis (cattle) swine herids disease (man) abortion, stillbirth (sheep) periodic ophthalmia (horse)
4. L. Grippotyphosa (Bovis)	Cattle, swine	Still birth (swine) infection haemoglobin urea Reproductive failures (cattle)

Transmission:

1. Contaminated pasture and water with infected urine, faeces, aborted foetuses and uterine discharge.
2. Through coitius and artificial insemination.
3. Abrasion of skin.
4. Man contact with infected animals.
5. Organism resist pasturisation and thrive in the soil for more than a year.

Symptoms and Lesions: *Cattle:*

A. Acute form:

1. High temperature.
2. Septicemia with petechiae on all visible mucous membranes.
3. Haemoglobinemia, Anaemia and jaundice.
4. Liver showed haemorrhages near central vein.
5. Kidneys are swollen, red.

B. Sub-acute form:

1. Mild to acute form.
2. Icterus may not be seen.
3. Interstitial nephritis with infiltration of lymphocytes and plasma cells.
4. Foetus in advance putrifaction.
5. Placenta is retained always.

Sheep and goats:

1. The disease is per acute.
2. Symptoms and lesions : As in cattle
3. Nervous form (shifting gait) may be seen in more acute form.

Pigs:

1. Abortion and or birth of weak piglets.
2. Focal intestitial nephritis.

Horse:

1. Conjuntivitis, keratitis and photophobia.
2. Abortion, Icterus and haemoglobenuria.

Dogs: Acute form:

1. Icterus, dehydration, vomiting and bloody diarrhoea.
2. Increased E.S.R.
3. Albiminuria.
4. Striking lesion are seen in liver, petachial haemorrhages, liver cells shrinky, dissociation from cards, focal liver cell necrosis.
5. Bile canaliculi are plugged and bile retained.
6. Kidneys show visible petachial haemorrhages.
7. The convoluted tubules severely affected the epithelium disquamated, swollen, coursely granular and deeply eosinophilic.
8. Lymph nodes and spleen, enlarged and haemorrhagic.
9. Diffuse haemorrhages are common in the fundic portion of gastric mucosa.
10. Haemorrhages on mycocardium urinary bladder, adrenal-glands, pancreas, gall bladder and lungs.

Sub-Acute:

1. The animals die form uremia.
2. Dehydration, emaciation, and strong uremic smell.
3. The renal lesions are more significant—the kidneys are

grossly enlarged, surface smooth, small haemorrhages.

4. Convoluted tubules undergo degenerative changes with accumulation of chronic inflammatory cells.
5. Glomeruli do not show changes.
6. Lesion in other is due to uremia-gastric haemorrhages caloaereous deposits in the wall of aorta and large arteries.

ULCERATIVE LYMPHANGITIS

It is a chronic contagious disease of horse mainly, may affect, cattle, caused by corynebacterium pseudotuberculosis (ovis), a gram positive, pleomorphic, non-sporulating organism.

Transmission:

1. Wound infection of the hind limbs.

Lesions:

1. The organisms enter the lymphatics and along the course of the lymphatic abscess is formed.
2. This abscess open up the discharge into a thick creamy pus which is blood stained.
3. The ulcers have a rugged appearance, which heal leaving a scar.
4. Regional lymphnodes are not affected.

Diagnosis:

1. Lesions
2. Demonstration of organisms.

BOVINE LYMPHANGITIS

It is an infectious disease of bovines with abscess formation in superficial lymph glands. It is caused by pasturella pseudotuberculosis rodentia type-III.

Transmission:

1. Wound infection most common.
2. Blood sucking insects (ticks, mites & fleas) transmit the disease.

Symptoms:

1. Prescapular precrural lymphnodes enlarged.
2. Affected limb shew lamenes.
3. Extension of infection to lungs through emboli cause pneumonia.

Lesions:

1. Lymphangitis and lymphadimitis.
2. Abscess from the lymphatic system, emitting white, thick and granular pus.
3. Suppurative pneumonic lesions.

Diagnosis:

1. Smears form pus reveal bipolar organisms.
2. Straus test: Male G. Pig 1/p inoculation with organisms causes suppurative orchitis.

MYCOPLASMOSIS

In this chapter infectious agent involved in contagious bovine pleuropneumonia and contagious caprine plurophenmonia are described.

The organisms show brownian movement under light microscope. The organisms are plemorphic with no definite cell wall. They form elongated branching shape in which may be seen ovoid to round structures which give the filament a beaded appearance.

Genus and Species	Disease
Mycoplasma mycoides V.Mycoides.	Bovine pleuropneumonia
Other bovine mycoplasmoses	
M. agalactiae V.bovine.	Mastitis
M. Bovigenilaticum	Seminal vesicultis and epi demitis.
M. Bovoculi	Infectious bovie kerato conjunctivitis
M. Bovirhinis. M.dispar.	Enzootic pneumonia of calves
M. Mycoides. V. capri	Contagious caprine pleuropneunonia.
M. agalactiae	Contagious agalactia of sheep and goats
Other mycoplasmoses in goats and sheep	
M.ovipneumoniae M. arginini.	Pneumonia
Mycoplasma sp. Mycoplasma sp.	Arthitis, pleuritis and pericardtis kerato conjuntivitis
M. Hyosynoviae M. hyorhins	Mycoplasma arthritis and polyarthitis in swine.

CONTAGIOUS BOVINE PLEUROPNEUMONIA

This is highly infectious disease of cattle caused by M. Mycoides. Bison, buffalo, yak, reindeer and antelopes which are rarely affected. [Calves under one year of age are less susceptible.]

Transmission:

1. Droplet infection.
2. Closed housing, transport may favour early infection.

3. Contaminated food and water through nasal discharges milk and urine.

Incubation period: 3 weeks to 6 months.

Pathogenesis:

1. Organisms enter the bronchioles via the respiratory tract set inflammation of bronchiolar wall.
2. Passes through the wall into the interlobular septa causing inflammation of the lungs-croupus pneumonia.

Symptoms:

1. Painful cough, nasal discharges, characteristic rales.
2. Recovered animals are carriers-lungers.
3. Mucopurulent discharge form the nose.
4. The organisms passes through placenta resulting in abortion.
5. Oedema infiltrating the lower thorax.

Lesions:

1. Lesions are limited to one lung.
2. Plural cavity contains excess fluid which is serofibrinous.
3. On section lungs show marbled appearance—Red and greyish areas of parenchyma separated by thick yellow interlobular septa.
4. Thrombosis of the branches of pulmonary arterines leading to necrosis of lungs—such necrotic areas are separated from healthy areas from—sequestra.
5. Internal organs showed degenerative changes.

Diagnosis

1. Based on symptoms and lesions
2. Demonstration of organisms.

3. Complement test for confirmation
4. Slow inoculation of lymph from the affected animal into calf results large edimatous swelling locally.

CONTAGIOUS CAPRINE PLCUROPNEUMONIA

It is a serious respiratory disease of goats caused by Mycoplasma mycoides var capri causing heavy mortality.

Transmission:

As in CBPP.

Incubation period: 8-28 days.

Pathogensis & symptoms :

As in CBPP.

Lesions:

1. Catarrhal inflammation of upper respiratory tract.
2. Lungs uniformily consolidated with fibropurulent exudate on pleura.
3. Pericarditis is frequent.

Diagnosis:

1. Based on symptoms and lesions.
2. S/c inoculation of lymph into healthy goats results in oedimatous swelling following death.
3. Demonstration of organism.

DIFFERENTIAL DIAGNOSIS

	CBPP	CCPP
1.	Cattle usually affected	Goats are usually affected.
2.	Disease is subacute/chronic	More acute
3.	Involvement of upper respiratory tract - less	Mostly affected.

4.	Pneumonic lesions diffase	Foecal.
5.	Marbling of lungs—prominent	Less prominent.
6.	Sequestratum is characteristic feature	Not a feature
7.	Pericaronditis not common	Common
8.	Exudate in chest is less and does not clot.	More and tends to clot on exposure to air.

2

VIRAL DISEASES

Foot and Mouth Disease

(Aphthous fever)

It is a contagious disease of cloven footed animals, caused by epitheliotropic- entero virus of the picarna group. Cattle and pigs are mostly affected, less of sheep and goats. Wild ruminants may be affected (reindeers, antelope, deer). Horses not susceptible. Camels, lab animals and man are susceptible.

Serotypes:

Seven immunologically different types were recognised. Strain, A.O.C., SAT (South African—strain) 1,2,3 and ASIAN -1.

Incubation period : Few hours to few days.

Rout of Infection:

1. Ingestion—contaminated food and water—The virus is discharged through saliva, semen, urine, Faeces and milk).
2. Mechanically—Man and other animals.
3. Aerogenous—Virus present in saliva even before vesicles form.

Pathogenesis:

Virus invades the epithelial cells (gastric, intestinal) multiply and produce focal areas of degeneration and inflammation. Cells undergo vacculation, pyknosis of nuclei and losening of cell connection together with leucocytic infiltration. The virus enter the lymph and blood and reaches the epithelium of mucous membrane and skin producing vesicles.

Symptoms:

1. High fever (104-106°F), anorexia, depression. The temperature falls on the formation of vesicles.
2. Vesicles are seen on tongue, mouth, feet and teats.
3. Saliva dribbling.
4. Vesicles rupture and form angry ulcers with rugged and irregular borders.
5. Eating difficult with mouth lesions.
6. Walking difficult due to foot lesions.
7. Milking difficult due to lesions at the orifice of teats.
8. Secondary complications develop due to contamination of wounds.
9. Animal lose condition rapidly and become emaciated, period of convulsion is long.
10. Because of endocrine involvement, recovered animals have dry and rough coat with long hair—such animals are called panters.

Lesions:

1. Mostly squamous epithelium is affected—tongue, buccal mucosa, rumen, reticulum, omasum, skin of udder, teats, coronary bands, conjunctiva.
2. Vesicles are seen on the dorsum of the tongue (anterior 2/3 and lateral aspects)—lips, cheek, gums, dental pad and hard palet.
3. Gastroenteritis.
4. Sucking calves die due to gastroenteritis, before vesicle develops.

5. Respiratory symptom—Catarrhal inflammation, oedema of lungs and sub-pleural haemorrhages.
6. In severe cases heart is affected dilated and flabby. Ventricle muscle, septal wall of left ventricle and papillary muscle showed greyish streaks giving the heart a tigroid appearance (Hyaline degeneration).
7. Spleen may be enlarged and soft.
8. Cerebral ventricles contain abundant fluid.
9. The lesion in sheep and goat are similar but mild.

Diagnosis:

1. Based on symptoms and lesions.
2. The disease must be differenciated from vesicular stomatitis (affect horses), vesicular exzanthema (affects pig), rindeppest and mucosal disease.
3. Complement fixation test.
4. Virus neutralisation test.
5. Biological—G.pig inoculation with vesicular fluid in foot-pad-vesicles develop in 1-7 days. Vesicle appears after 1-2 days.

VESICULAR STOMATITIS

It is an infectious disease of horse, cattle and pigs. This disease has seasonal incidence and hence thought to be due to some insect vector-flies and mosquitos.

Incubation period: 24-48 hours.

Lesions:

1. Seen in oral mucosa.
2. Only in swine.
3. No myocardial lesion.

Diagnosis:

This disease can be produced in cattle by linqual rout only.

VESICULAR EXANTHEMA

It is an acute infectious disease of pigs. Laboratory animals are not susceptible. Infection is by ingestion of infected meat.

Incubation period: 16-28 hours.

Lesions:

1. Similar to foot and mouth disease.
2. Vesicles are found on the snout, nose, tongue, lips, gums, interdigital space, dew claw, coronasy band udder and teats.

Diagnosis:

1. Complement fixation test.
2. Virus neutralisation test.
3. Agargel diffusion technique.

Differential Diagnosis

	Cattle	Horse	Pigs	Sheep	G.Pig	Man
Foot and Mouth	+	-	+	+	+	+
Vesicular stomatitis.	+	+	+	+	+	+
Vesicular Ex-hanthema.	-	+	+	-	-	-

RINDERPEST (CATTLE PLAGUE)

Acute contagious disease of cattle, sheep and goats. The virus is immunologically and pathologically related to canine distemper and measles virus. The virus are attached to the leucocytes. The virus is found in blood during the height of fever and latter localises in spleen, lymph glands and liver mortality is 100%.

Incubation period:

i. Experimentally :- 2-3 days.

ii. Through Attendents : 6-9 days.

iii. Outside the body the virus cannot thrive more than 24 hours.

Pathogenesis:

The virus has got great affinity to lymphoid cells and epithelial cells of elementary tract. The nucleus undergo Pyknosis, Karyorexis, necrosis and finally Karolysis leaving reticular mesh alone.

The other cells present are plasma cells, macrophages. Such changes were found in lymphnodes, spleen, and patches.

Symptoms:

1. High fever, anorexia, lacrimation, dryness of muzzle.
2. Increased thirst.
3. Photophobia.
4. Mucopapular rash develops on those parts of body where there are no hair.
5. Severe abdominal pain.
6. Constipation followed by diarrhoea with fall in temperature.
7. Diarrhoea—very offensive in smell, faeces contain mucous.
8. Death in 6-12 days.

Lesions:

1. Lesions on the oral mucosa appear in 2 or 3 days after fever.
2. Ulcers are seen inside the lower lip, commsure of the mouth, under side of the free portion of tongue, fore stomach.
3. There are no vesicle formation due to the movement of the mouth, the necrotic tissue cast off leaving shallow erosions with raw red surface and sharply demarked edges.

4. Abomasum is always affected. Ulcers are severe at the pyloric region. Folds of abomasum are thick and edimatus and contents are chocolate in colour due to blood from the erosion. Stuffing of the mucous membrane.
5. Small intestine: Not severe as in abomasum and large intestine.
6. Duodenum and ileum, affected payer's patches are necrotic and shows deep ulcers.
7. Large intestine: Prominent lesions are found at Ileocaecal Junction and in rectum. These are as show diffuse haemorrhages, ulceration and pseudomembranes. These sheets of haemorrhages on the folds of mucous membrane of the rectum are responsible for the so-called Zebra markings.
8. Microscopically—Epithelium is shead, leaving the lamuna propria, which shows haemorrhages, oedema, leucocytic infiltration, multinucleated gaint cells contain eosinophillic cytoplasm. All these changes leads to thickness of the wall.

Sheep and Goats:

1. Dullness, diarrhoea, heavy mortality due to secondary penumonia are the symptoms. There are no mouth lesion, as they are found in cattle.

Rarely lesions are haemorrhagic in the respiratory mucosa, subpericardial, epicardial, in the bladder and vagina liver showed passive venous congestion.

Diagnosis:

1. Based on symptoms and lesions.
2. Compliment fixation test.
3. Agargel diffusion test.
4. Serum virus neutralisation test.

5. Intranuclear and intracytoplasmic inclusion bodies in the epithelium and lymphoid tissue.

MUCOSAL DISEASE

(Bovine Viral diarrohea)

It is a disease of cattle and buffaloes between 6-14 months of age. It is called mucosal disease, because it affects predominantly mucosa of the digestive tract. Mortality is high (100%) and mortality is low (4-8%).

Incubation period: 8-10 days.

Infection:

Ingestion of contaminated food and water.

Symptoms:

Mild form:

1. Slight temperature.
2. Leucopenia.
3. Diarrohea for few days.

These symptoms pass of unnoticed.

Acute form:

1. High fever.
2. Suddcn fall of milk.
3. Rapid pulse and depression.
4. Loss of appetite
5. Diarrohea is watery, profuse and foul smelling.
6. Cough increase respiration with mucous or meucopurelent nasal discharge.
7. Necrotic erosions may be seen on the mucosa of mouth, pharynx, skin and nose.

8. Severe bloody diarrohea.

This period lasts for 2-4 weeks.

Chronic form:

1. Intermittent diarrohea.
2. Gradual emaciation.
3. Cataracts, renal atrophy, micro-ophthelmia, optic neuritis, malformation of the choriocapillaries in calves born to infected dam.

Lesions:

1. Lesions confined to mostly mucous membrane of gastro-intestinal tract. The lesions are described as erosions of the epithelium leaving shallow ulcers. These lesions result from atrophic and cystic changes of the gastric glands. Oedema, congestion and occasional haemorrhage in lamina propria and submucosa.
2. Oral mucous membrane of tongue, gums, lips, cheeks, palate, pharynx and oesophagus showed erosions.
3. Haemorrhages on the leaves of omasum.
4. Small intestine: payers patches necrosis and sloughing of lymphoid tissue.
5. Caecum and colon:— Catharral inflamation, congestion, excess mucous, haemorrhagnes, ulceration and necrotic patches of the mucosa.
6. Petachae on caecum, haemorrhages in vagina and epicardium.
7. Lymphnodes of intestine:— Slightly oedema.
8. Retropharyngial lymphnodes—enlarged.

Diagnosis:

1. Based on symptom and lesions.

2. These disease must be differenciate form F & M and R.P.

Differential Diagnosis:

		F.M	R.P	M.D
1.	Animals affected	Cattle & Pigs mostly	Bovines, sheep & goats	Bovine only
2.	Age group	All the age groups	All the age groups	Younger groups 6-14 months
3.	Mortality	High	High	Low
4.	Morbidity	Low	High	High
5.	Lesions	Vesicles form	No vesicles Erosion usually, become ulcers and covered by bran-like deposits of flakes.	No vesicles, seldom become ulcers not covered by flakes.
6.	Payers patches`	Not affected	Necrosis & deep ulcers	Slight erosion occasional ulcers
7.	Large intestine	Slight congestion	Zebra markings	Congestion cattarhal inflamation.
8.	Lymphoid tissue	Nalesion	Severely destroyed & necrotic change	Only mild change

		F.M	R.P	M.D
9.	Mouth Lesion	All parts of mucous membrane of mouth and 1/3 and sides of tongue	Inner mucous membrane of lower lip and under surface of free portion of tongue.	All portions of the mucous membrane of mouth all over the tongue.
10.	Foot lesions	Present	Not present	Not present
11.	Stomach lesion	Lesion in rumen recticulum, omasum	Abomasum only near pyloric end.	Abomasum only near Fundus.

POX (VARIOLA)

It is an acute disease of cattle, horse, buffaloes, swine, fowls and man. The condition is malignant in sheep and many other species caused by dermatotrophic virus. The virus of human, bovine and equine strains are related.

Pathogenesis:

The Virus has special affinity for the prickle cell layer and passes through different stages.

1. Rosiolar stage—First there will be congested spots.
2. Papular stage—Initial proliferation of cells giving rise to small papules.
3. Vesicular stage—There will be swelling of cells and degeneration, increased inflammatory hypermia with severe exudation of epidermis and the cells detached to form vesicle.
4. Pustular stage—Leucocytes enter the vesicle and the cells get digested forming crest which may cast off.

5. Desquammation stage:— Pastules dries up forming a crest which may cast off.

The cutaneous lesions were found to be of three types viz diserete, confluent, haemorrhagic. The cutaneous lesion is a circumscribed zone of hypermia and lymphocytic infiltration in the dermal papillae underlying the affected epidermis. Cytoplasmic includes bodies in the affected cells-Borrel granules were found.

Incubation period: 2-3 days.

Infection: Through

(i) Attendants.

(ii) Contaminated milking machine.

(iii) Flies

(iv) Milkers nodules—dairy men who have contacted the pox nodules on their hands from the infected udder and teats in cows.

Cow pox (vaccine): Buffalo Pox is milder than vaccinia. Vaccina virus is used for immunisation against small pox in humans.

Horse pox: Milder, caused by vaccina virus. Lesions are seen on pastern, buccal meucosa and nostrils.

Sheep pox: Virus is host specific. Goats get milder attacks. Goat pox gives immunity against sheep pox, whereas sheep pox does not give immunity against goat pox. Sheep pox is severe with many fatalities. It is a generalised infection.

Swine pox: Cow pox virus affects and causes severe lesion in adults; swine pox virus affects piglets mostly.

Incubation period: one week.

Lesions:

1. In general the lesion are similar in all the species affected but the severity varies.

2. Initially there will be fever followed by nodular formation in hairless parts udder, teats, lips, eyelids, skin underneath the tail, vulva, scrotum and perpuce, trachea, pharynx.
3. The sheep pox vesicles are different from that of cow pox, the floor of the vescile in sheep pox is formed by Corium, while in cow pox is the stratum germinatum.
4. In papular stage the cells appear as histocytes. They are large cells with basophillic cytoplasm. The nuclei is oval or irregular with large nucleolus. The cytoplasm contains acidophillic-infected bodies.
5. Pharynx, trachea and abomasum-vesicles or ulcers.
6. Other lesions include, fatty degeneration of parenchymatus organs, petchiae on serous membranes and interstitial nephritis.

Diagnosis:

1. Based on symptoms and lesion.
2. Demonstration of intracytoplasmic granules.
3. Gelprecipitation test.
4. Serum neutralisation test.

SWINE FEVER (HOG CHOLERA):

It is caused by filtrable virus, associated with secondary infection with bact. cholera susis, past septica and many others. Pigs of all ages affected, but older ones suffer mildly.

Infection:

1. Ingestion through contaminated food and water (virus is discharged through urine, blood, saliva)
2. Inhalation.
3. Conjunctive and nasal mucoses.
4. Recovered animals are carriers.

Incubation period: 6-9 days.

Pathogenesis:

Virus gain entry into blood through tonsils, multiply rapidly in blood leading to septicemia. The virus affects primarily endothelial cells causing haemorrhages, necrosis and infection in various organs.

Symptoms:

Peracute:

Found in young pigs, disease develops rapidly and terminates fatally in three days.

Acute form:

1. The course is slower and death occurs in 1-2 weeks.
2. High temperature (106°F) and loss appetite.
3. Severe leucopenia, total WBC count will be less than 4,000/-cmm.
4. Conjunctivitis with thick sticky discharge.
5. Nervous symptoms are frequent, lethargy, occasional convulsions, grinding of teeth, and difficulty in locomotion.
6. Skin—Erythmatus lesions in the abdomen, axilla, inside the thigh.
7. Intestinal and pulmonary involvement is frequently noticed.
8. Early pregnancy infection, results in embryonic death and abortion.
9. Infection in late pregnancy results in mumification, ansarca, ascities, still birth with cerebellar hypoplasia, lymphomyelino genesis, congenital tumors and neonatal death.
10. Chronic form— Not commonly recognised, unthriftness. Affected pigs survive.

Lesions:

Vary greatly in individual pigs, but depends upon the severity of the infection.

A. Peracute form: There are no lesions.

B. Acute Form: Numerous puntiform or large haemorrhages will be seen in skin, various organs and subcutaneous tissue. Diffused congestion of inflammation of the mucous membrane of stomach, small intestine and occasionally large intestine.

3. Petechial haemorrhages are found in small intestine, peritonial surface, pericardium and endocardium.
4. Petechial haemorrhages in the context of the kidney gives a characteristic, appearance-turkey egg marking when the capsule is removed.
5. Spleen may be enlarged and show haemorrhagic infarcts.
6. Mesentric lymph glands enlarged, congested with haemorrhages.
7. Lungs showed numerous small haemorrhages all over the surface and consolidation.
8. Mucous membrane of bladder showed haemorrhages.

Chronic Form:

1. Intestine:— Characteristic ulcers seen in small intestine mostly at illiocaecal valve and the first portion of large Intestine. Also epiglottis, tongue, pharynx, larynx, stomach, and occasionally in the skin of yearlings.
2. Ulcers consists of circumscribed areas of necrosis of grey, yellow or black colour, which usually contain a series of concentric rings. In early stages the lesions are more or less flat, but in older ones ulcers are prominent called Button ulcers.
3. Endothelium of blood vessels and capillaries swollen with hyaline degenerations, haemorrhages, thrombi and infarcts

in various organs, perivascular cuffing present.

Diagnosis:

1. Symptoms.
2. Typical P.M. lesions.
3. Inoculation in young G.P., typical lesion produced with leucopoenia.
4. Acute Arteritis.
5. Fluoroscent antibody technique.

INFECTIOUS CANINE HEPATITIS:

(Rubarth diseases, Hepatitis contagisal canis)

It is a acute viral disease of dogs. Young dogs suffer more. The virus is identical to pox encephalitis virus.

Infection: By ingestion of contaminated feed and water.

Incubation period: Few hours to few days.

Symptoms are:

A) Per acute.

B) Acute

A. Per acute:

1. Animal dies within 12-48 hours with slight interus.

B. Acute:

1. If the animal is serviced for 24 hours, recovery occurs within 4-10 days.
2. High temperature, salivation, anorexia and thirst.
3. Sub-cutaneous oedema of head, neck, and abdomen.
4. Vomition with bloody diarrhoea.
5. Clonic spasms of the extremities, neck, paralysis of hind

quarter.

6. The mucous membrane showed icterus.
7. Petachiae on gums.
8 Keratocongentivitis of one or both the eyes and corneal opacity.
9. Tonsil enlarged and congested.
10. Increased albuminusia.
11. Neutropoenia, lymphocytopoenia initially followed by lymphocytosis.
12. Prolonged bleeding time.
13. SGPT and SGOT found levels increased.

Lesions: A. Per acute.

1. Tonsils and lymphonodes of the entire body enlarged and congested.
2. Haemorrhages of meninges, spinal chord, brain, thymus, heart, stomach, and intestine.
3. Serosanguinus fluid and abdominal cavity.
4. Liver enlarged, congested with focal necrosis.

B. Acute:

1. Endothelial and hepatic cells are mostly affected leading to necrosis.
2. Histologically hepatic cells lose the staining affinity, the nuclei are not visible, sinusoidal endothelium swollen with enlarged pyknotic nuclei.
3. Basophilic intranuclear inclusion bodies are found in the endothelial cells, hepatic cells and kuppffer cells.
4. The wall of gall bladder is thickened.

5. Acute gastero enteritis, and pancreatitis.
6. Kidneys:— Intranuclear inclusion bodies are found in endothelial cell of glomeruli and occasionally in the epithelium of collecting tubules.
7. Spleen:— Enlarged due to engorgement. Intranuclear inclusion bodies were found in the reticuloendothelial cells.
8. Brain:— Haemorrhages in thalmus, midbrain and medulla and oblongata.

Diagnosis:

1. Symptoms and lesions.
2. Demonstration of intranuclear inclusion bodies.
3. Severe hypoglycemia.

CANINE DISTEMPER

(Hard pad disease, carries disease)

It is caused by pantropic virus. Characterised by diphasic fever, acute catarrhal inflammation of mucous membranes, pneumonia and pustule formation under the abdomen and thigh. Young dogs and under one year of age suffer more.

Infection:

1. Ingestion of contaminated food and water.
2. Inhalation.
3. Secondary infection with bronchiseptica in pneumonic lesion and with salmonela species in gastric lesion is always common.

Incubation period: Five days.

Pathogenesis:

From the site of entry the virus is carried to the regional lymphnodes. Where they multiply and enters the blood leading to virmia. Finally the virus settles and multiply in the epithelium of skin, G.I tract, respiratory, urinary and biliary tract. Also multiply in the nuclei and cytoplasm of neurons and ganglion.

Symptoms:

1. Diphasic fever, nasal discharge and conjunctivitis.
2. Brainchitis, pneumonia, cough and dyspnoea.
3. Pustules on the lower abdomen and inside thigh due to the invasion by pyogenic bacteria.
4. Diarrhoea and dehydration.
5. Eye:— Keratitis, retinitis and blindness.
6. Nervous system:— epileptic seisures excessive chewing.
7. Hyperkeratosis of digital pad-hard pad disease.

Lesions:

1. Respiratory lesions are most common in majority of the cases. There will be purulent bronchopneumonia. The lesions initially catarrhal followed by purulent seen in nose, pharynx, larynx and bronchial mucosa.
2. G.I. Tract: —The lesions are acute catarrhal type. Payer's patches and solitary follicles show congestion and swelling.
3. Spleen slightly enlarged.
4. Large quantities of pericardial blood accumulation, fatty degeneration of cardiac muscle.
5. Kidneys and liver show parenchymatus degeneration.
6. Congestion and haemorrhages of meninges and brain: Non-supprative encephalitis.
7. Intracytoplasmic or intranuclear inclusion bodies are seen in the epithelial cells or mucosa of nose, pharynx, urinary bladder, bile duct, genital passage.

Diagnosis:

1. Symptoms and lesions are diagnostic.
2. Demonstration of intracytoplasmic and intranuclear acidophilic inclusion bodies.
3. Ferret innoculation.
4. Florescent antibody technique.

RABIES

(Hydrophobia, Lyssa)

It is a neurotroplic viral disease of all warm blooded animals including man, affecting the C.N.S.

Infection:

1. Bite of rabid animal
2. Contamination of water with infected saliva.
3. Insectivorous and fungivorous bats, harbous and virus.
4. Vampire bats are important in spread of the disease to animals and man without showing any clinical symptoms.
5. The virus present in the saliva of dogs five days before clinical symptom are manifested.

Incubation period:

It depends upon the site of the bite. The nearer the bite to the head the shorter the incubation period. This varies form 2-7 days.

Pathogenesis:

Virus reaches the brain from the site of infection through nerves or blood. Multiply in ganglion cells and spread through nerves to the salivary glands. The virus present milk and spread to the foetus through placenta.

Two types of viruses noticed viz

1. Street virus is the virus which is found in naturally infected

cases.

2. Fixed virus: If the street virus is passaged through rabbit innoculation for fifty time, it becomes fixed properties of reproducing the disease and incubation period.

The difference between:

	Street Virus	**Fixed Virus**
1.	Incubation period is variable.	It is fixed.
2.	Intracerbral inocuation of rabbit, death results in 14-20 days..	Death results in 7 days.
3.	Negribodies are present.	Absent
4.	Salivary glands affected.	Not affected.

Symptoms:— are seen in two forms.

a) Dumb form

b) Furious form

a. Dumb form: The animal is more comatose with vacant looks. Sit in corners, does not obey master with lower jaw hanging.

b. Furtus form: The animal is very excitable, bites on everybody indiscriminately, barks at immaginary objects, chews all sorts of objects (sticks, stones), drinks its own urine, champing of jaw, and walk miles.

Paralysis follows in both the forms leading to death in 7-10 days.

In cattle and sheep bellowing and in horses colic are important symptoms. Bulls and ram show excessive sexual urge.

Lesions:

1. Seen in C.N.S. only, which includes hypermia, oedema of meninges with petchiae.

2. Microscopically non-suppurtive encephalitis, perivascular cuffing.

3. Babes nodules: Foetal proliferaton of satellite (microglia) cells around ganglian cells, with mild infiltration of lymphocytes and plasma cells.

4. Changes are most frequent in hipocampus, the brain stem and gassarian ganglian.

5. Acute catarrh of the mucosa of respiratory and G.I. tract, fullness of gall bladder, hypermia of kidneys, spleen and liver.

6. Negribodies: These are inclusion bodies found in the cytoplasm of neurons. They are round with clear hallow around. These bodies are acidophilic containing basophilic granules.

Diagnosis:

1. Symptoms.

2. Suspected dog must be isolated for ten days. In rabies, dog dies in seven days.

3. Impression smears of hipocampus major. Negribodies can be demonstrated with manns stain.

4. Rabbit inoculation into brain.

5. Complements fixation test.

6. Fluorescent antibody test.

AUJESZKY'S DISEASE

(Pseudorabies, Infectious bulbar paralysis, Maditch)

It is caused by pantropic virus belonging to Herpes virus group. Many species of animals including man are susceptible.

Infection:

1. Pigs and rodents are the natural hosts.

2. Rubbing on an abraded snout of pig.
3. Intranasal inoculation.
4. Ingestion of infected food and water.

Incubation period : 7 days.

Symptoms:

Cattle:

1. Violent itching of the part.
2. High fever, paralysis and death within forty-eight hours.

Pigs:

1. Paralysis and inco-ordinate convulsions, tremors and vomiting.
2. Pruritis absent.
3. Death within twelve hours after onset of symptoms.

Lesions:

1. Localised inflammation and oedema of the infected part.
2. Inflammation of respiratory and G.I. tract.
3. Necrotic foci in spleen, liver and heart.
4. Inclusion bodies Intranuclear found in degenerated neurons.

Diagnosis:

1. Symptoms.
2. Subcutaneous inoculation of infected material in the rabbit pruritis within 48 hours and dies with tonic spasums.
3. Fluorescent antibody technique.
4. The disease must be differentiate from rabies.

	Rabies	Pseudorabies
1.	I.P. Long	Short (24-48 hours)
2.	Course upto 10 days	2 days
3.	No itching	Itching present
4.	Consciousness lost	Not lost
5.	Inclusion bodies intracytoplasmic	Intranuclear
6.	S/c inoculation into rabbit; Infection does not occur	Infection occurs.

BLUE TONGUE IN SHEEP

(Catarrhal fever of sheep, "Sore muzzle")

It is a viral disease of sheep, causing mortality 50% and morbidity 7%. The virus belongs to orbivirus. The disease is severe in sheep and milder in cattle, goats and deer.

Infection:

1. Culicoides, biting insect transmit the disease.
2. Melophagus ovinus mechanically transmit the disease.

Incubation period: 5-7 days.

Pathogenesis:

Blood vessels are affected leading to hypermia, oedema and haemorrhages in all the tissues. Haemopoitic tissue affected resulting in anaemia and leucopenia.

Symptoms:

1. High temperature of 105°F and associated symptoms.
2. Edimatus swelling of lips, tongue and face.
3. Oedema and cyanosis of tongue known as blue tongue disease.

4. Petchiae on oral and nasal mucosa.
5. When the temperature comes down, flushing of the skin and feet appears.
6. The caronet becomes warm and tender and later the pink perioplic band turns red.
7. Haemorrhages into the medullary canal of the growing horn at the junction of the skin and hoof-streaky zone, parallel to periople.
8. Finally severe emaciation, prostration and muscular weakness (occassionally torticollis), penumonia and death.
9. In prolonged cases a break on the growth of wool may cause the fleece to be shed.

Lesions:

1. Changes in the vascular system-Arteritis-severe engorgement of blood vessels, endothelial hyperplasia, and infiltration with neutrophils, lymphocytes in the adventisia of the oral mucosa, brain, placenta.
2. Tongue and check-hypermia, oedema, cyanosis, multiple haemorrhages finally leading to erosions and ulcers.
3. Skin-hypermia and the subcutis particularly around the head and neck is edimatus.
4. Musculature-foci of haemorrhages and necrotic changes in muscle bundles, hyalinisation.
5. Digestive system-bleeding from the mucosa of abomasum and deudenum, liver showed fatty change in periportal zone.
6. Pericardial sac filled with blood tinged fluid.
7. Lungs edimatus and poneumonic.
8. Spleen enlarged and slightly congested.
9. In sheep infected in 4-8 weeks pregnancy-lambs may be

stillborn or dummies. Animals walk aimlessly by circles, buts against objects and do not nurse unless helped.

Diagnosis:

1. Symptoms.
2. Lesion.
3. Isolation and identification of virus.
4. Serum neutralisation test.

EPHEMERAL FEVER

It is a viral disease of cattle of three days duration with no mortality.

Infection:

1. Virus is associated with leucocytes and platelets, hence infection is due to inoculation.
2. Development of virus occurs in insects (sand flies-ceratopogo midae species)

Incubation period: 10-20 days.

Symptoms:

1. High temperature which returns to normal in three days, with associated symptoms.
2. Animal is stiff with tremours and returns to normal in 3-5 days.

Lesions:

1. After initial virimia the virus localised in joints, lymph nodes and muscles.
2. Serous cavities contain increased amount of fluid together with congestion or petachial haemorrhages.

Diagnosis:

1. Three days sickness and quickly returning to normalcy.

CONTAGIOUS ECTHYMA

(Pustular dermatitis, sore mouth)

It is a disease of sheep and goats caused by dermatotrophic virus. Lesions are usually found on the lips and udder. Man contact the disease.

Infection:

1. Virus are found in scales viable for 15 days.
2. Contacts.
3. Contamination of wounds.

Incubation period: 5-8 days.

Symptoms:

1. Congested areas were seen first on the skin at the corners of the mouth and lips.
2. These later develops into papules, vesicles and finally pustules.
3. Pustules dry forming yellowish scabs.
4. Mouth lesions causes difficulty in feeding.
5. Udder lesions leads to mastitis.

Lesions:

1. Lesions are similar to pox viz. papule, vesicles, pustules and finally scab formation.
2. Secondary lesions lead to complication like matitis.

Diagnosis:

Based on symptoms & lesions.

AFRICAN HORSE SICKNESS

(Equine plague, lapesteducheval)

It is a highly fatal disease of horses, mules and donkeys caused by viscerotropic virus. Virus seen in tissues and fluids in the body. Mortablity 90%.

Infection:

1. Bitting by gnat-culicoides.
2. Dog is reservoir for the virus.

Incubation period: 5-7 days.

Symptoms:

(A) Acute pulmonary form (DUNKOP):

1. Most common.
2. Sudden rise in temperature with concomitant respiratory symptoms.
3. Pulmonary oedema, nasal discharge, profuse swetting.
4. Death in few hours.

(B) Sub-acute cardiac form (DIKKOP):

1. Fever develops slowly and lasts longer.
2. Characteristic oedema of head (temporal fossa), lips, eyelids, neck and chest.
3. Tongue swollen, cynotic with petchiae on the ventral surface.
4. Paralysis of oesophagus—difficulty in swallowing.
5. Cardiac failure—pulmonary edema—hydropericardium and endocarditis.
6. Mortality high due to pulmonary form.
7. Death due to cardiac failure.

(C) Mild form

1. Initial rise of temperature which returns to normal within 1-3 days.

2. Anorexia, dyspnoea and mild conjunctivitis.
3. Mortality varies 25-90%.

Lesions: Pulmonary form:

1. Hydrothorax, usually accompanied by severe oedema of sub plural, interlobular stroma and fills alveoli in many lobes.
2. There is leucocytosis with Bronchopneumonia.

Cardiac form:

1. Hydropericardium with petechae and inflammatory oedema in epicardium.
2. Myocodial necrosis, haemorrhages.
3. Lymphopoenia is evident in spleen and lymph nodes.
4. Oedema around pharynx might be due to paralysis of oesophagus.
5. Haemorrhages in gastric mucosa and pelvic fat of kidneys.

Diagnosis:

1. Based on symptoms and lesions
2. Intracerebral inoculation of mice.
3. Virus neutralisation test.

EQUINE ENCEPHALOMYELITIS

It is a disease of central nervous system of mainly horse, caused by virus of different strains, viz Western strain, Eastern and Venezuelon. It is not recorded in India.

It is transmitted through mosquitoes. The affected animals wanders aimlessly, walks in circles. High temperature when nervous symptoms appear, temperature returns to normal. There is facial paralysis and unable to stand. Mortality varies 50 - 90%.

The lesions are mainly present in C.N.S and neurons. Various degenerative changes leading to necrosis, perivascular cuffing.

Intra-nuclear acidophilic inclusion bodies in the neurons present.

DIAGNOSIS is made:

1. Based upon symptoms and lesions
2. Isolation and identification of virus by Rabbit or G.Pig inoculation.

EQUINE INFECTIOUS ANAEMIA

It is a viral disease of mainly horses, transmitted through the bite of mosquitoes and flies.

The disease runs into three stages, viz., 1) Acute 2) Sub-acute and 3) Chronic form, but difficult to differenciate. The symptoms are rapid high fever (108°F) with associated symptoms, anaemia, oedema of dependent parts, pale mucus membrane. Low R.B.C. count (1.5 million/Cu.mm). The animal is thin inspite of good appetite.

Diagnosis is based upon symptoms, gel diffusion test and fluorescent antibody test.

3

DISEASES CAUSED BY PROTOZOA

COCCIDIOSIS

They are intracellular parasites of intestinal epithelium. Coccidia belongs to the class sporozoa. The two pathogenic genera are Eimeria and Isosopra. They affect animals and birds. The following species affect different animals.

	ANIMAL	SPECIES	LOCATION
1	Cattle	E.Zurini E. Bovis E.Ellipsoidalis	Caecum, colon Terminal portion of Ileum small intestine
2	Sheep and goat	E.Parva E.Arloingi E.Fauri	Small intestine
3	Dog & cat	I. Bigemina I.rivolta I.Felis I.canis	Small intestine
4	Swine	E.debleiciki I.suis	Small intestine
5	Fowl	E.Tenella E.Necatrix E. burnetti	Caceum, small intestine and caeeum
6	Rabbit	E.Stieda	Intrahepatic bile duct
7	Geese	E.truncata	Renal tubules.

Infection:

1. Ingestion of contaminated food and water.
2. The oocysts containing sporocysts (four oocyst with two sporozoites in Emieria and two oocyst with four sporozoites in Isopora) are ingested.

Pathogenesis:

The life cycle is divided into a sexual phase and asexual phase.

Asexual phase: In the ingested oocyst the sporzoites mature and on release invade the intestinal epithelium and develop to become mature trophozoites (G. Schizonts). Each mature schizont contain numerous merozoites, which affects the new epithelium again. They develop into new schzonots containing again merozoites (2nd generation).

Sexual phase: The second generation merozoites enters into new epithelial cells, develop themselves into male (microgametocytes) and female (macrogamitocytes). The microgramtocytes penetrate the mature macrogamitocytes to form zygote covered with thick wall—very resistant and variable for two years in unfavourable conditions.

During the development of these parasites, there is heavy destruction of intestinal epithelial cells, leading to haemorrhages and anaemia.

Diagnosis:

1. Symptoms and lesions.
2. Presence of oocyst in faeces.

BABESISIS

(Piroplasmosis, tick fever)

It is a protozoan disease of animals. The parasite inhabit the R.B.C. consisting of binary fission. The sexual life cycle occurs inside the tick which is the intermediate host.

Infection:

1. By a bite of tick.
2. Transplacental—Rare
3. Inoculation of infected blood.
4. Transmission can be from stage to stage—Nymph stage is infected it becomes adult and pass on infection to adult.

Cattle	B. Bigemina.
	B.Bovis
Sheep & Goat:	B.Motassi
	B.Ovis
Horse:	B. Equi
	B.caballi
Dogs:	B.Canis
	B.Gibsoni

Incubation period: 1-4 weeks.

Pathogenesis:

The organisms proliferate by bending a reduced form of schizogony forming pairs. During this process the red cell breaks. The parasite when liberated attacks fresh RBC's.

Symptoms:

1. Calves under six months of age are resistant.
2. High fever 104-106°F, conjunctive is highly injected.
3. Haemoglubinmia in the urine is black coloured.
4. Blood is watery.
5. Musosa pale, anaemia progressive, dyspnoea develops followed by Icterus.

6. Anorexia, depression and stopage of rumination.
7. Decreased milk yield.
8. Pregnant animals abort.
9. Ascites may develop in some cases.
10. Death in 10-12 days.
11. In acute phase the organism found in peripheral blood of erythrocytes. The infected erythocytes are bigger than the normal erythrocytes.
12. Reduction in total RBC's count, haematorit and haemoglubin values.
13. Blood changes—Anisocytosis, poikilocytosis, puntate basophilia followed by normoblasts.
14. Bone marrow hyperplastic.
15. Sheep and goat—The symptom are less severe.
16. Horse (biliary fever) trasmitted by rhipicephalus evertsi, R. Bursa, Dermacentor and Hyalomma. The symptoms are as described above but mortality is less.
17. Dogs (tick fever, Malignant jaundice)—B.Camis-transmitted by Rhipicphalus sanguineious a three host tick. B.gibsoni transmitted by Hemophysalis-bisipinosa a three host tick)

Symptoms are similar to cattle.

Lesions:

1. Carcass emaciated.
2. Petechial haemorrhages on the serous membrane, under cardiac serosa, mucosa of stomach and intestine.
3. Fluid accumulation in pertoneal and pericardial sacks.
4. Lungs edimatus.
5. Gastroenteritis.

6. All organs Icteric.
7. Spleen enlarged and the pulp is dark red in colour.
8. Liver enlarged and showed fatty changes with centrilobular necrosis.
9. Gall bladder distended with yellow granular bile.
10. Kidneys dark red, tubular epithelium showed degenerative changes and the lumen contains casts and haemoglobin.
11. Bladder contains blood-stained urine.

Diagnosis:

1. Examination of stained blood smears for protozoa.
2. Blood changes: Decrease PCV, ESR and haemoglobin.
3. Symptoms and lesions.
4. Carrier animals may be diagnosed by animal inoculation.

TRAYPANASOIASIS

It is a group of diseases affecting mammals, domesticated and wild, as well as man and birds. Among these diseases surrah is very important in India.

Various species and the diseases:

T- Evansi - Surrah in horses.

T-Equiperdum - dourine.

T- Brucei - Nagana or Tsetse fly sickness.

T-Equinum- Malde caderas.

T-Congolense- wasting disease in cattle.

T-Vivax - -do-.

T-Hippicum - parani

T-Cruzi - chagas disease in children.

T-Gambiense - sleeping sickness in man.

SURRAH

It is an acute or chronic disease of all domestic animals chiefly equines, caused by T.evansi. Horses, mules, donkeys camels, cattle, dogs and elephant are affected naturally. Sheep and goats rarely get the disease.

Infection:

Vectors - tabanus, stomaxys and hematopota transmit the disease.

Incubation period: Few days to three weeks.

Symptoms: May be acute or chronic.

Horses and mules:

1. Temperature rises 104-106°F.
2. Fever intermittent.
3. Urtricarial erruptions.
4. Frequent relapses of temperature.
5. Watery nasal discharge.
6. Oedema of the lower parts of the limbs extending later to the other dependent parts—throat, breast, belly, sheath and scrotum.
7. Weakness, staggaring gait finally leading to paralysis.
8. Pregnant animals abort.

Sub-acute or chronic form:

1. There is dullness.
2. Intermittent fever.
3. Wasting and anaemia.
4. Tenderness on loins and back.
5. Oedema of legs.

6. Ulcerative keratitis.
7. Diarrhoea.
8. Finally prostration and death.

Lesions:

1. Emaciation of carcass.
2. Enlargement of spleen.
3. Serous exudate in serous cavities.
4. Petachieal haemorrhages on serous cavities.
5. Congested areas in stomach and intestine.

Diagnosis:

1. Symptoms and lesions.
2. Demonstration of trips in peripheral blood smears.
3. Mercuric chloride test: Mix one drop of serum with ice of one in 25,000 solution of mercuric perchloride in water. In positive cases a white precipitate appears within few minutes.
4. Formal gel test: mix 2 drops of formaldehyde with ice of serum. After 24 hours a complete gelation is positive. It is only 75% accurate.
5. Complements fixation test.
6. Biological test: 2 cc of infected blood inoculated into rabbit or mouse. After a few days it can be demonstrated in blood.

LEISHMANIASIS

Bovines and dogs are affected and rarely seen in horses, goats and sheep. The disease is seen in three forms in man.

1. **Visceral form**: caused by leishmania donovani (kalaqzar), present in India, it may be acute or chronic.

Acute:

1. Fever, loss of weight and anaemia.
2. Enlargement of spleen, live and lymph-glands.
3. Ascitis and paralysis in few cases.
4. Leucopoenia.
5. Lesions: Intestinal ulcers, cloudy swelling of kidneys and strawberry colour of bone marrow.

2. **Cutaneous form:**

1. Caused by L.tropica—oriental sore or Delhiboli.
2. The organisms enter the skin by the bite of vector.
3. The organisms multiply in macrophages and liberated, which are ingested by other macrophages.
4. A papule formed due to the infiltration of neutrophils, lymphocytes and plasmacells.
5. The skin becomes hyperkeratotic and acanthotic on face, ears mouth and nasal cavity.
6. Sometime these lesions ulcerate.

Diagnosis:

Smears prepare from the spleen, bone marrow and skin stained with Giemsas, leishman-Donovan bodies can be seen.

AMOEBIASIS

Amoeba are unicellular organisms. E.histolytica is pathogenic and found in man and dog. In man it causes dysentery and abscesses of liver and in dog only dysentery.

Infection:

1. Through contaminated food and water.
2. The organisms remain without showing symptoms as carries, is a constant source of infection.

Pathogenesis:

The organisms have a thick cystic wall, which protects from the environment. This cyst is dissolved in intestinal juice, on ingestion and liberate four trophozoites. They divide to form eight amoebae. These secrete the proteolylic enzyme, which dissolves the epithelium of the intestine and facilitate penetration. In the intestine these amoeba multiply by binary fission.

The organism destroys crypts and superificial epithelium but not the muscular mucosa. The inflammatory reaction is minimal because the destruction is chemical in nature. The trophozoites may enter the circulation and reach the liver producing abscesses. Embolic abscesses may be found in liver and brain. The organisms encyst in the bowel before being discharged.

Diagnosis:

Demonstration of the organisms containing 1-4 nuclei in the feaces.

Index